A Great Body At Any Age
BODYMAGIC
Super-Gran Legs & Abs Routine

Julie & Gary Walsh

For the women that treasure their body as the precious gift that it is.

BODYMAGIC - Books By The Same Author.

A Man's Search For Meaning - *Identity Construction Of A Bodybuilder.*

Bodymagic - *Different For Girls*

Bodymagic - *A Beginners Guide To Training & Nutrition*

Bodymagic - *3 Legs & Abs Blasts*

Bodymagic - *3 Pecs & Lats Routines*

Bodymagic - *3 Upper Body Routines*

Bodymagic - *Fitness Facts*

Bodymagic - *Super-Gran Legs & Abs Routine*

Bodymagic - *Super-Gran Arms Routine*

Bodymagic - *A Physique Guide For Self Reliant Women*

Bodymagic - *A Physique Guide For Self Reliant Men*

Getting Better 1 - *Moving In The Right Direction - Ego Busting & Enlightenment In The Real World.*

Bodymagic - *Peak Contraction*

Contents

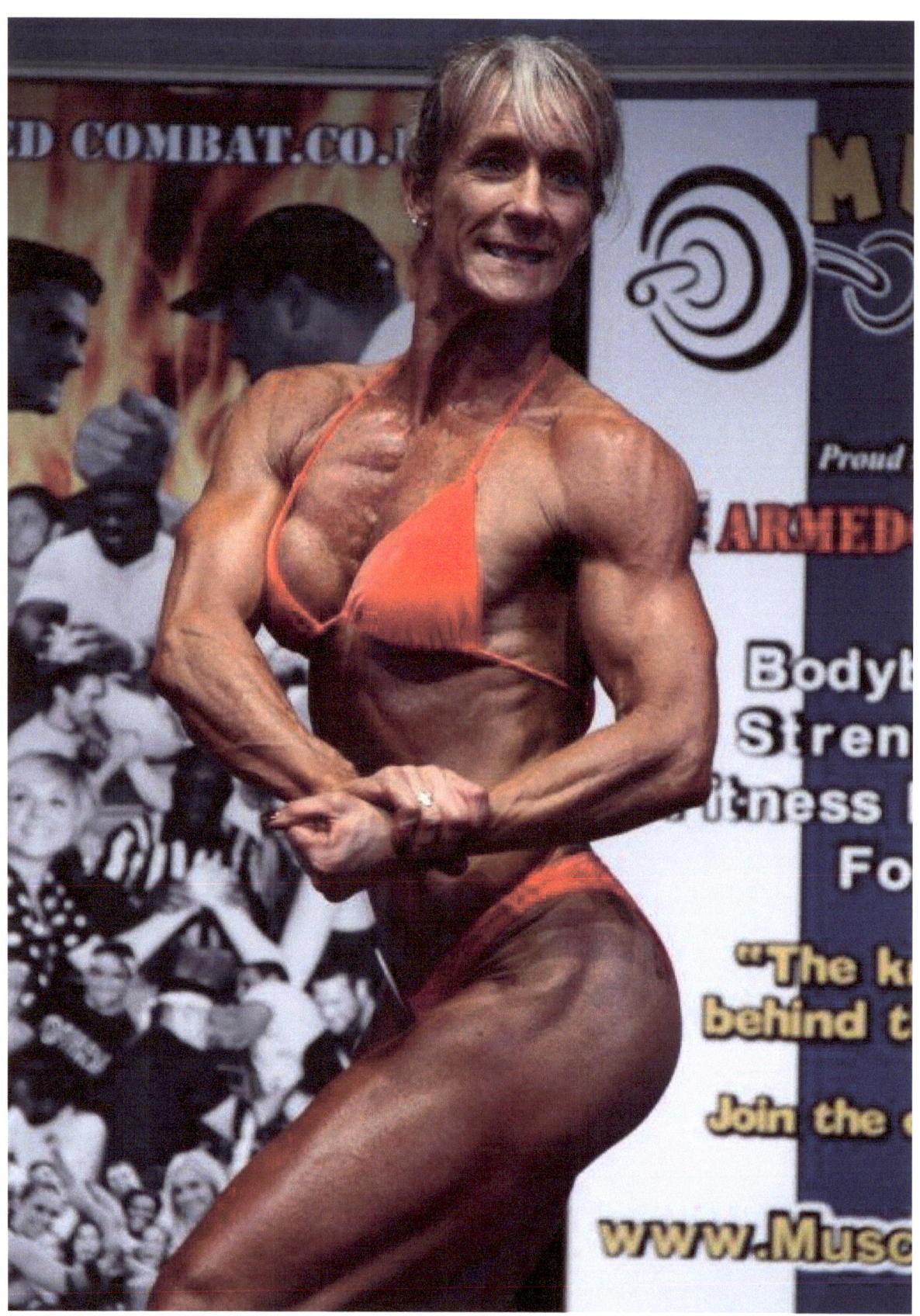

Super-Gran's Secrets

I have been married to Julie for 30 years now and I am probably the person best equipped to look at why she is able to stay in such good shape. There is really nothing super or special or even any secrets. Or maybe it is the mundane behaviours that make someone stand out in the 21st century. Julie eats well most of the time because she likes to and does not see it as a sacrifice. Julie never places limitations on herself as to what she can and cannot do. She never over analyses any situation as that can often lead to more reasons not to do something than give reasons to take on challenges. She also discounts many of the myths surrounding the fitness industry and prefers to try things for herself with a good positive headset. For Julie actions are what physique and fitness are all about. Stop all the planning and get on with it. Julie's pet shrug is listening to gym experts with theories and ideas but not realising that they are in the gym and now is the time for actions not words. I suppose if there is a secret it is to get on with the reason you are there when you are in the gym. Too often trainers have all the theory right but never ever train hard enough to see it through. They seem to think that the secret is in the theory. They would be better served to have no theory but just work hard and see results. To steal the slogan from Nike - "Just do it". Or what we like to say - "Get in - Work Hard - Get Out". It is not so much what you do as how you do it. This is true throughout life not just in the gym.

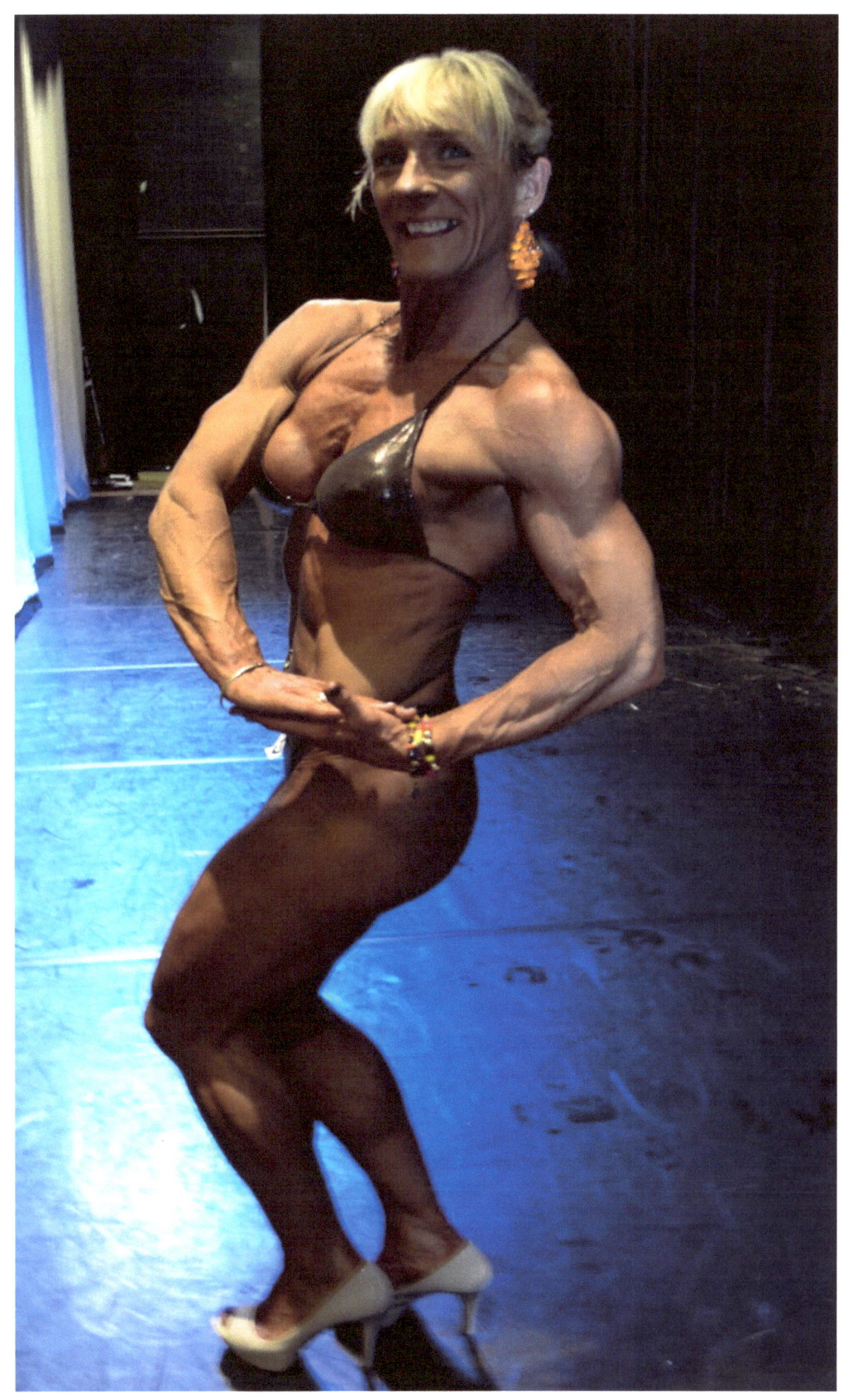

Introduction

It my intention here to give the reader just a small insight into the leg and ab exercises that I use on a regular basis and how I sometimes group them together for optimum results.

Leg workouts are a particular favourite of mine. The exercises that I list here are all used in preparation for shows and just generally when training for fun and maintaining in the off season. To be quite honest I never have an off season. I like to be in good shape all year and just step it up a notch just prior to any competitions. I am a physique girl 365 days a year not just for shows. I enjoy the gym and I enjoy training. I love the camaraderie and the physical and mental challenge that staying i shape has become in the land of plenty. To supplement my gym session I ride my bike to work(12 miles) and walk miles in nature with Gary and the dogs each week. We made the decision to get rid of the car at the same time as we got rid of our television so we could spend our time more productively with more activity including walking and maybe help the planet a little into the bargain. You would be amazed at how many people find it hard to relate to our voluntary simplicity, offering us lifts and enquiring how we can exist without the metal boxes in our lives. Gary has even dispensed with his phone. Severing attachment to these objects is not something we have regretted. In fact non-attachment is something we always look to do anytime we feel we are dependent on anything to the degree that its loss would feel catastrophic to us. To get back to the point - all the walking and biking I am now doing from breaking dependency on the gadgets is great for my legs and my fitness. I work abs and calves with my quads, hamstrings and glutes. The following is one quite unusual session that Gary put together for some variety to our leg workouts. I love the break from the norm that Gary's knowledge and imagination gives to our routines. We never do the same workout twice or at least that is how it seems.

1. Weighted Sit Ups

I like to begin with weighted sit ups on a leg day to hit my abs hard and heavy with a compound exercise which also works my hip flexors in readiness for the quad work to come. I feel these tie the abs and hip flexor area in nicely giving a look of unity as opposed to isolating and having the look of lots of separate bits. I go heavy. Gary hands me the weight discs and we normally only do 3 sets. With good diet and selective exercises one doesn't have to do endless ab exercises. They are worked indirectly throughout all sessions and as such only need a small amount of specialist work to keep them tight. Your diet and activity levels will unearth the hidden treasure.

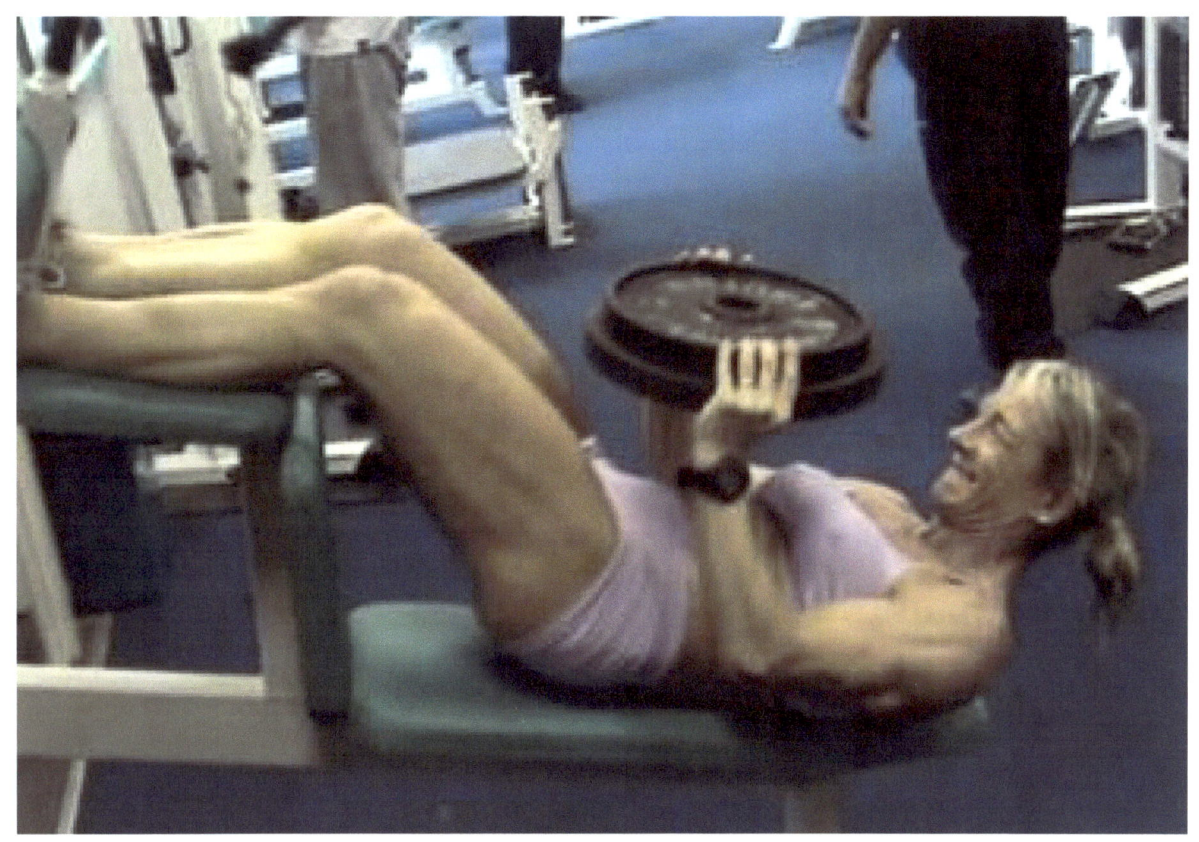

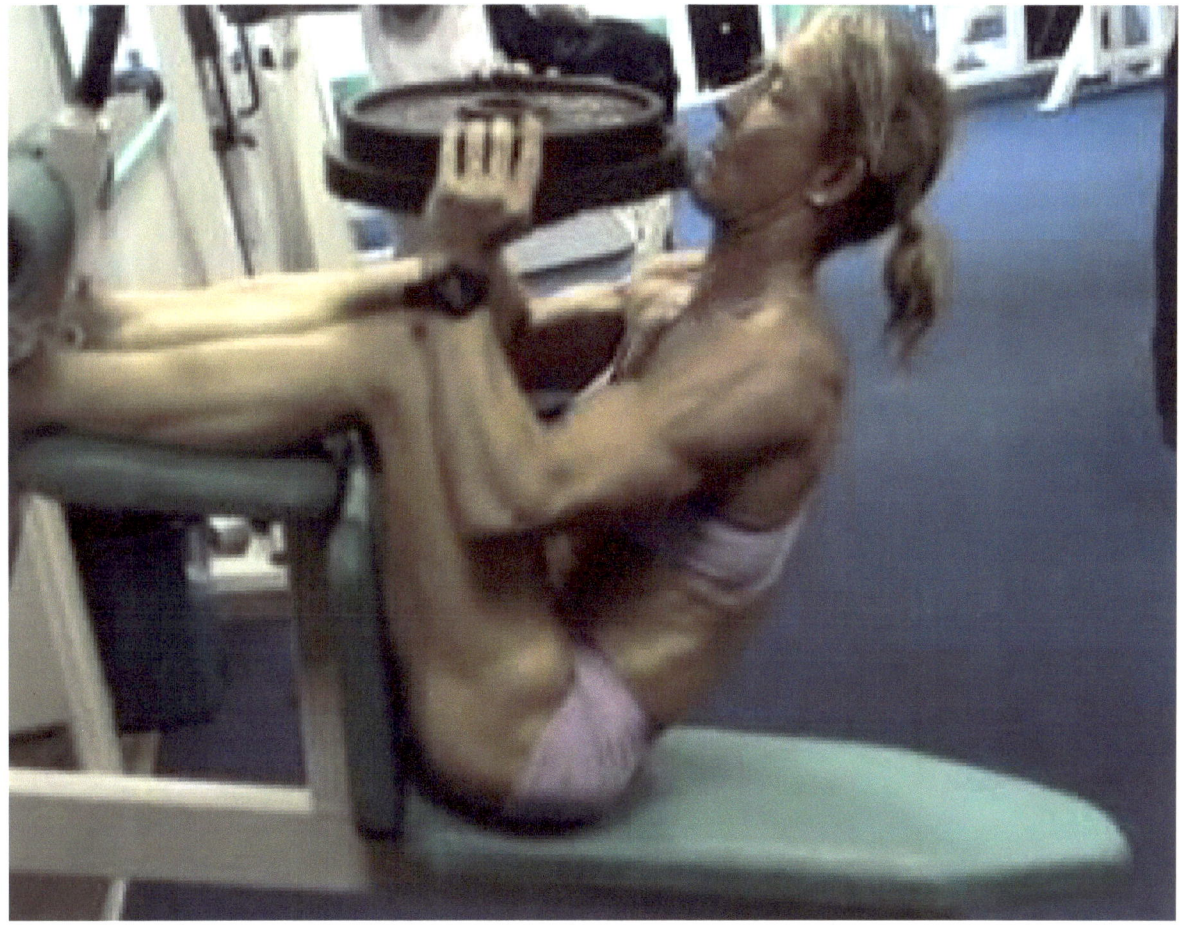

2. Seated Calf Raises

I like to do calves next in this session while my energy is high as too often calves are left until last as they are small and eventually they get left behind completely in favour of the larger more showy muscle groups. I also like to vary the reps from 12's up as high as 20 and above. Normally at least 5 sets. Often the last set is a strip down set. Working until failure and then taking off some weight and continuing. Two strip downs normally suffice. My calves are generally on fire by that time.

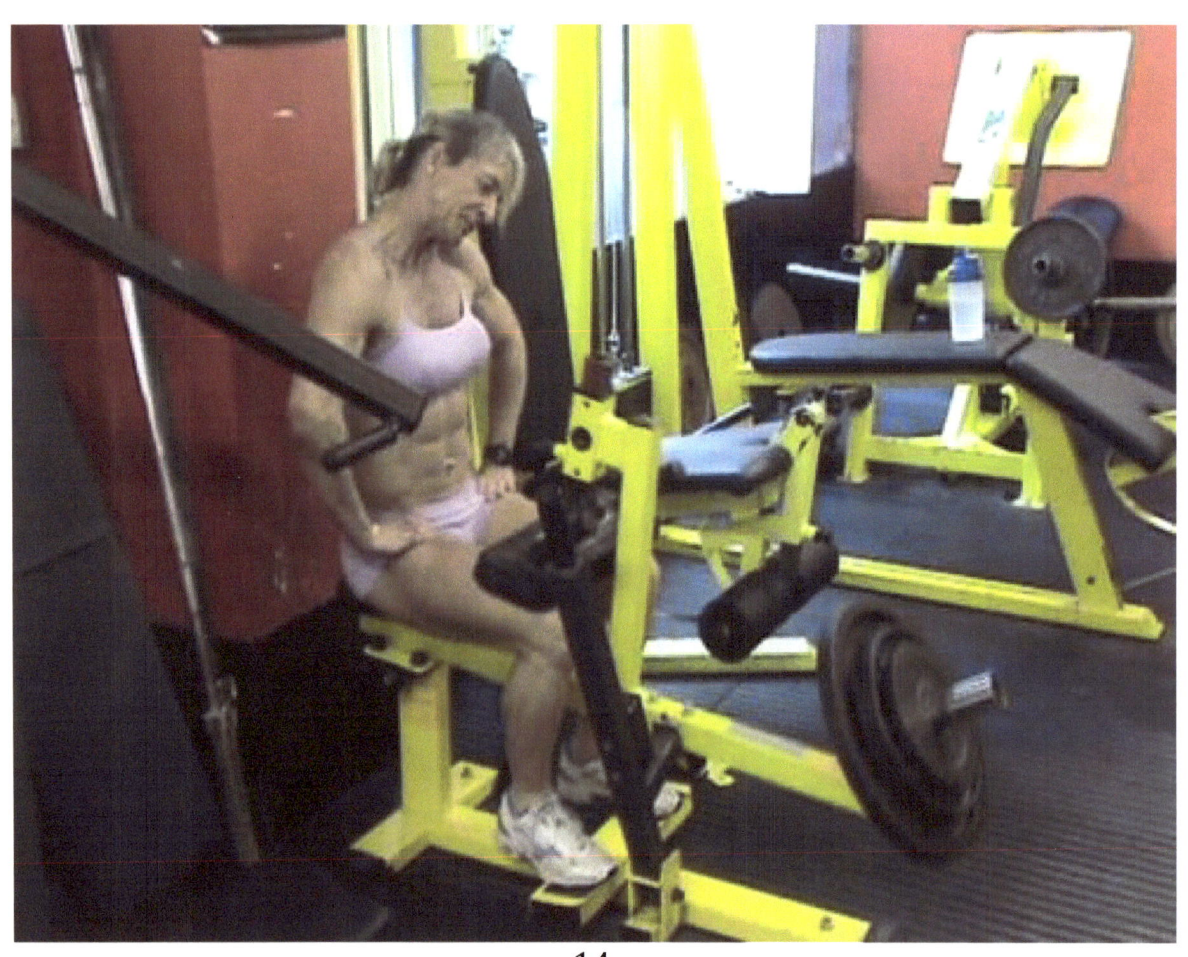

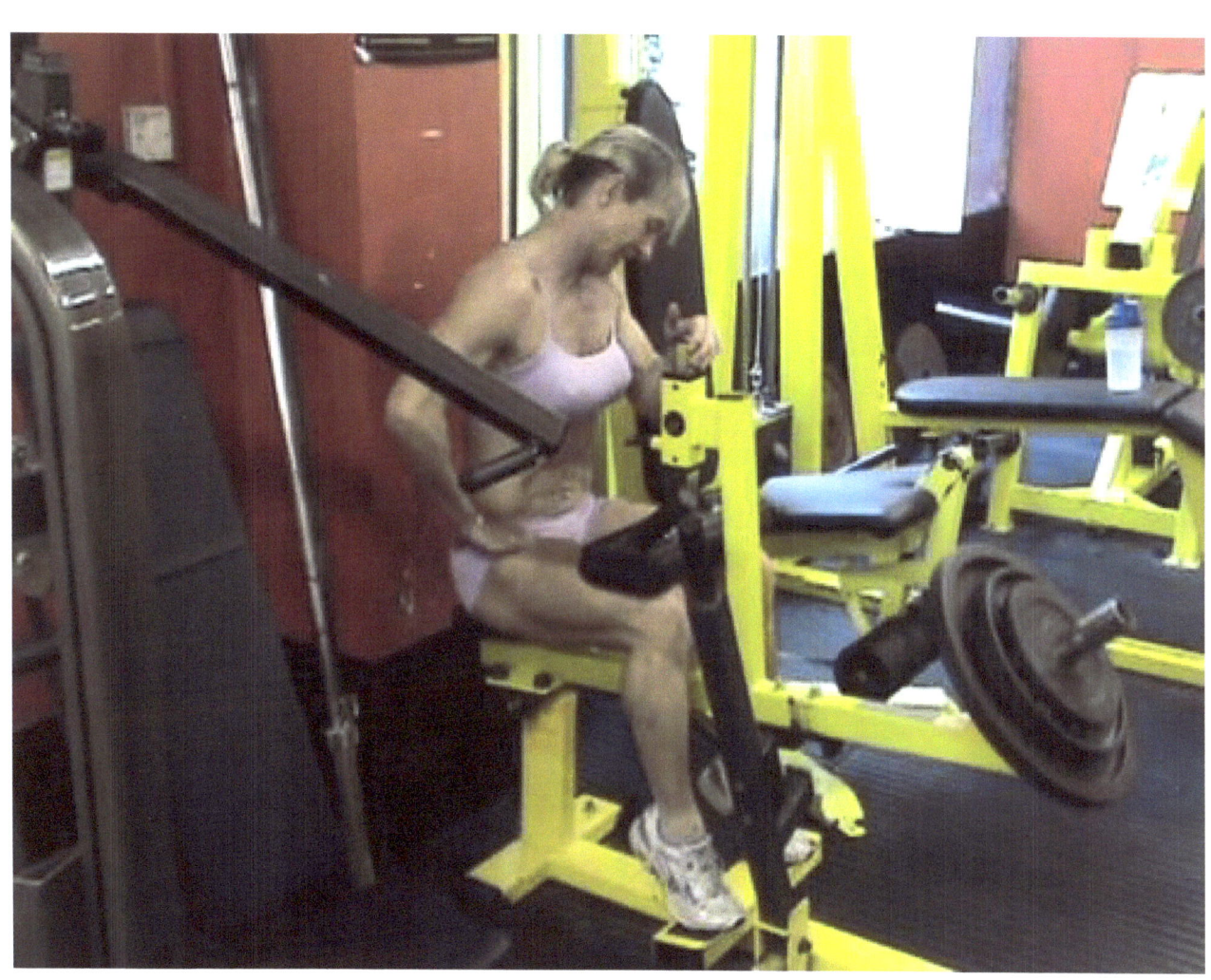

3. Standing Leg Curl & Bodyweight Lunges

There are 6 supersets in this combination. Three supersets with each leg. It goes as follows. I first do one set of leg curls with my right leg and with no rest immediately perform a set of bodyweight lunges again with a right leg lead. Next, I do the same with my left leg. I continue until I have done three with each leg. I do 12/15 reps and keep good form.

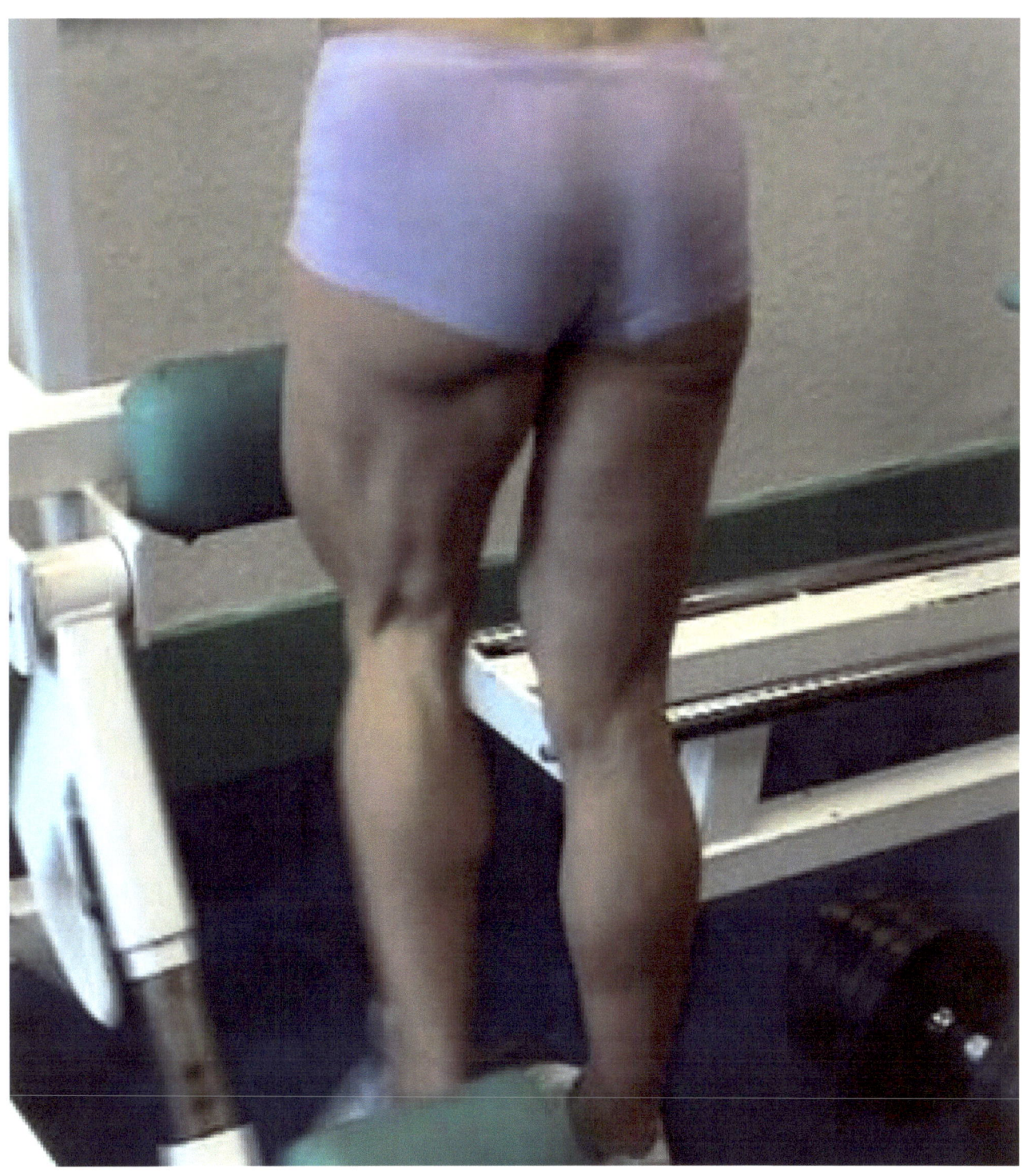

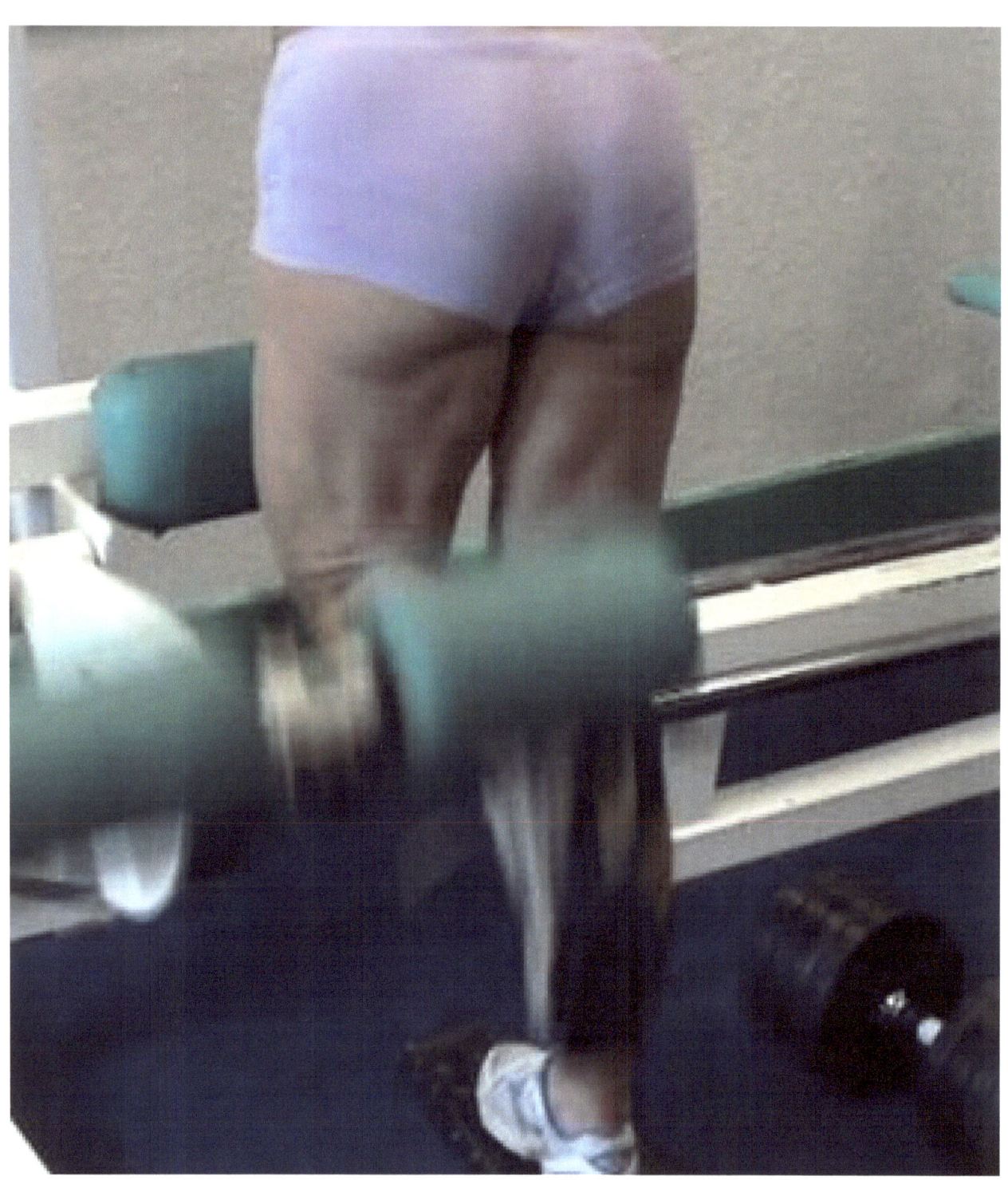

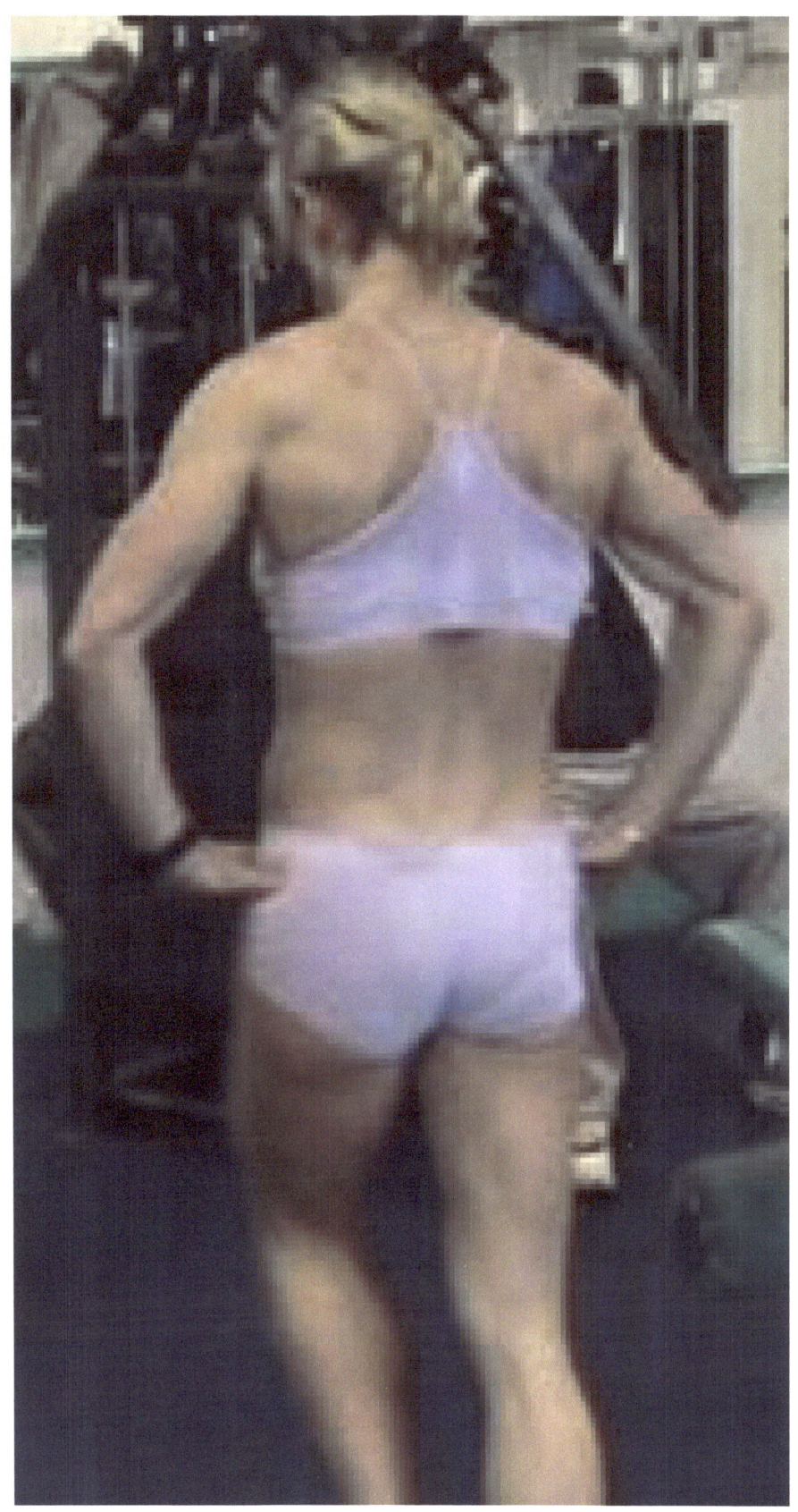

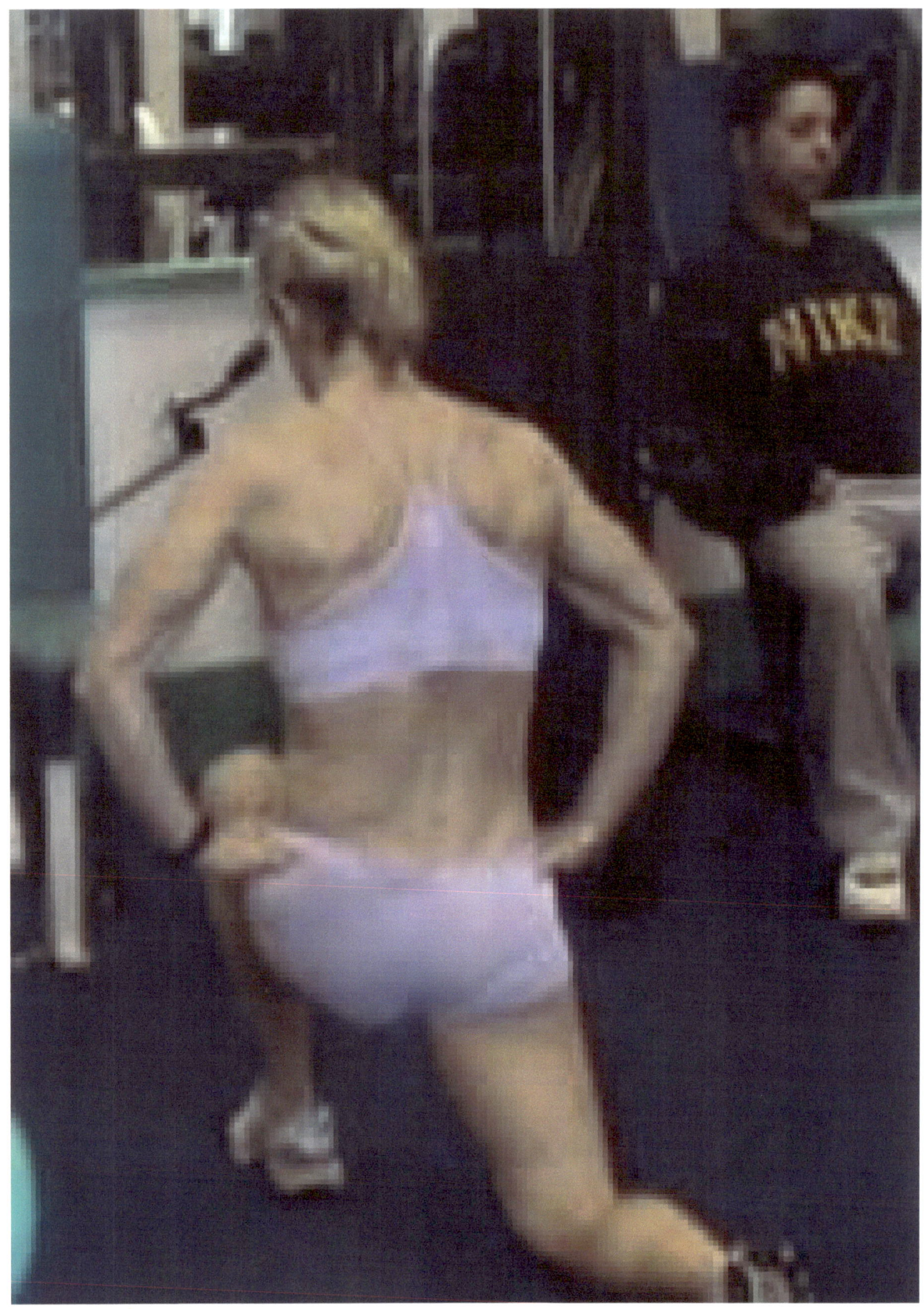

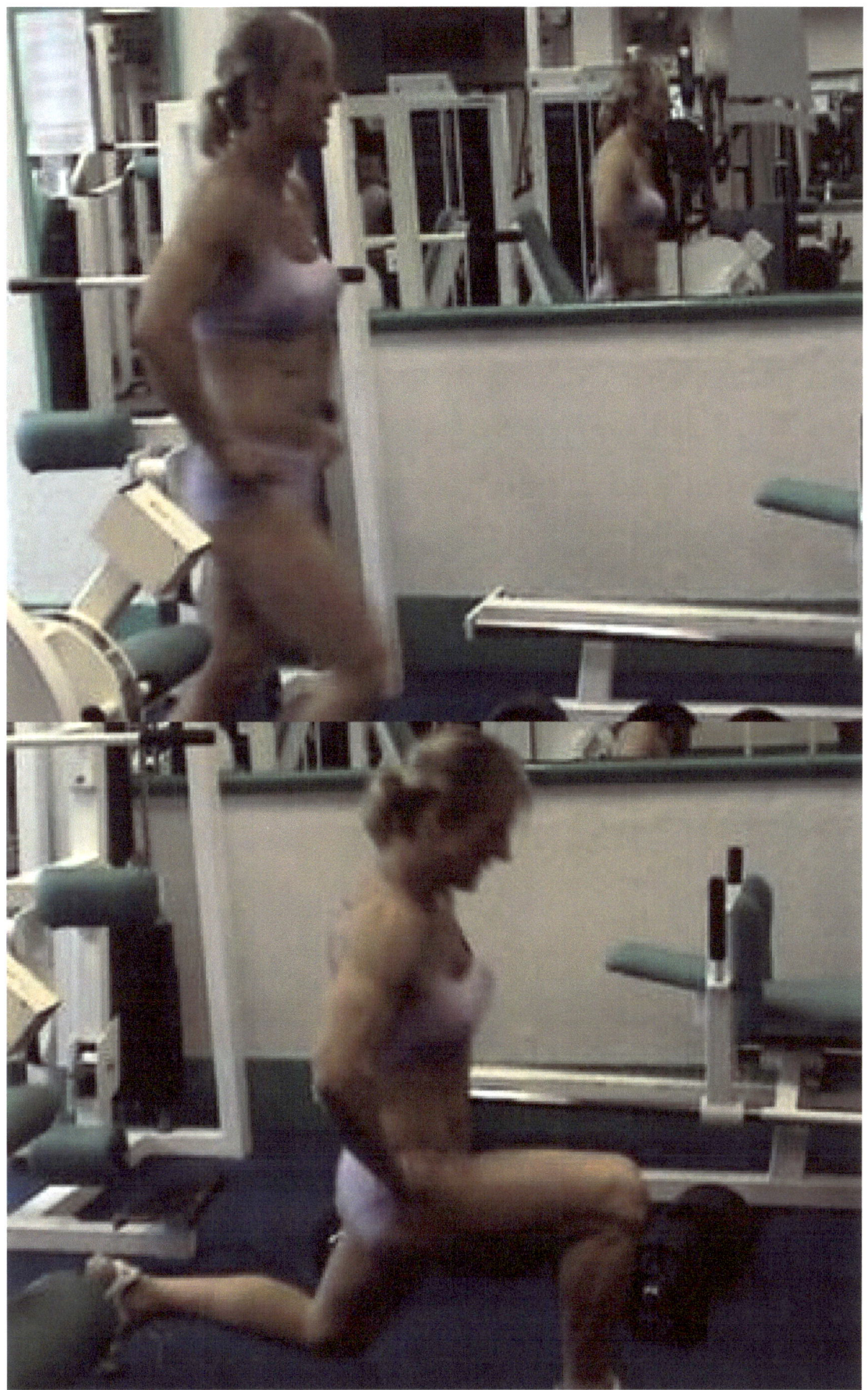

4. Single Leg Extensions & Split Lunges

Now I move to work primarily the quads although the hamstrings and glutes will still get some extra work from the split lunges. I will pre-exhaust the quads with leg extensions in a similar manner to the last combination. Working each leg three times in total as I am already well warmed up. This time I will use weight for the lunges and I will stay split throughout the entire set. I will not step forward each time. The pictures will show this clearly.

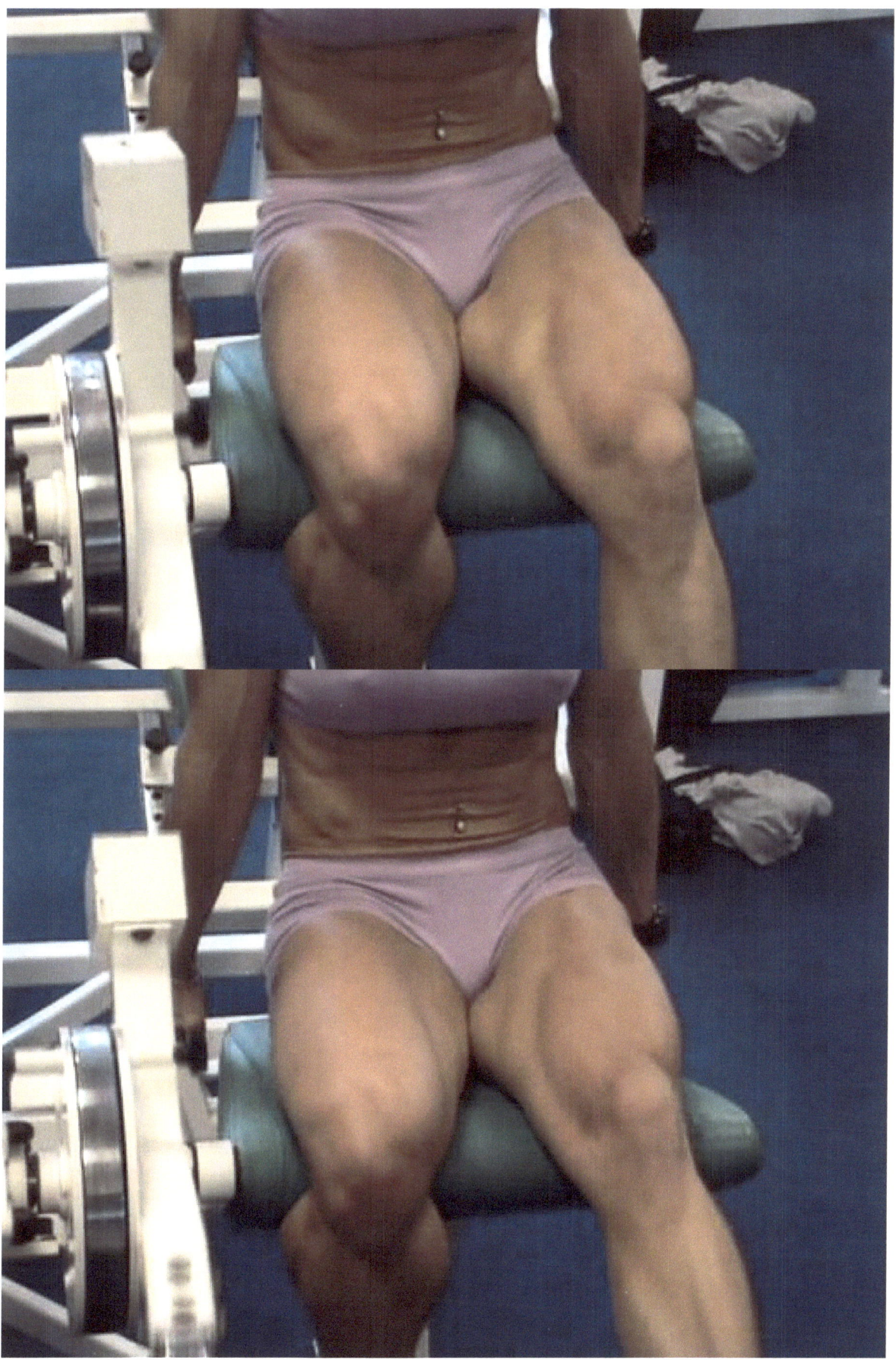

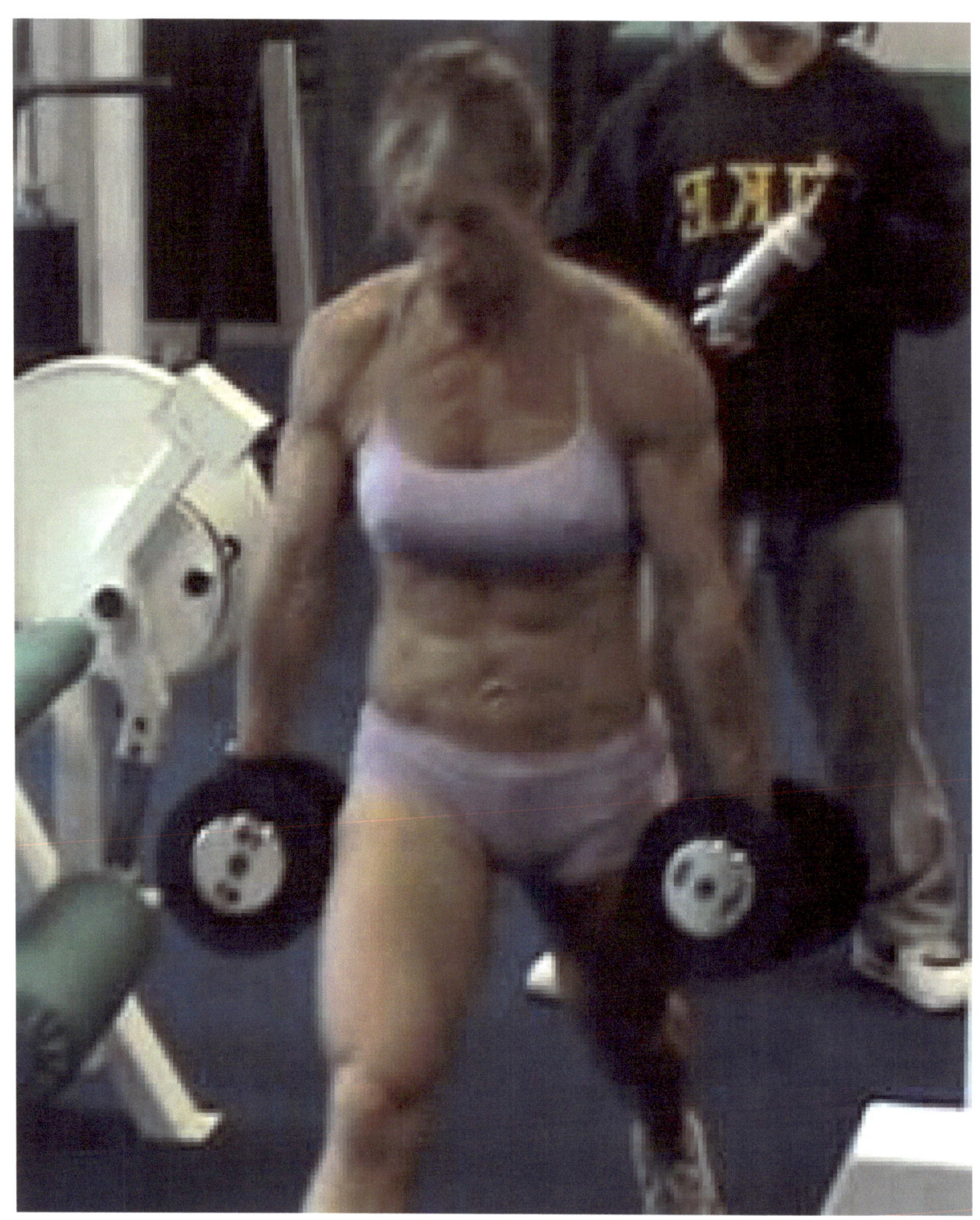

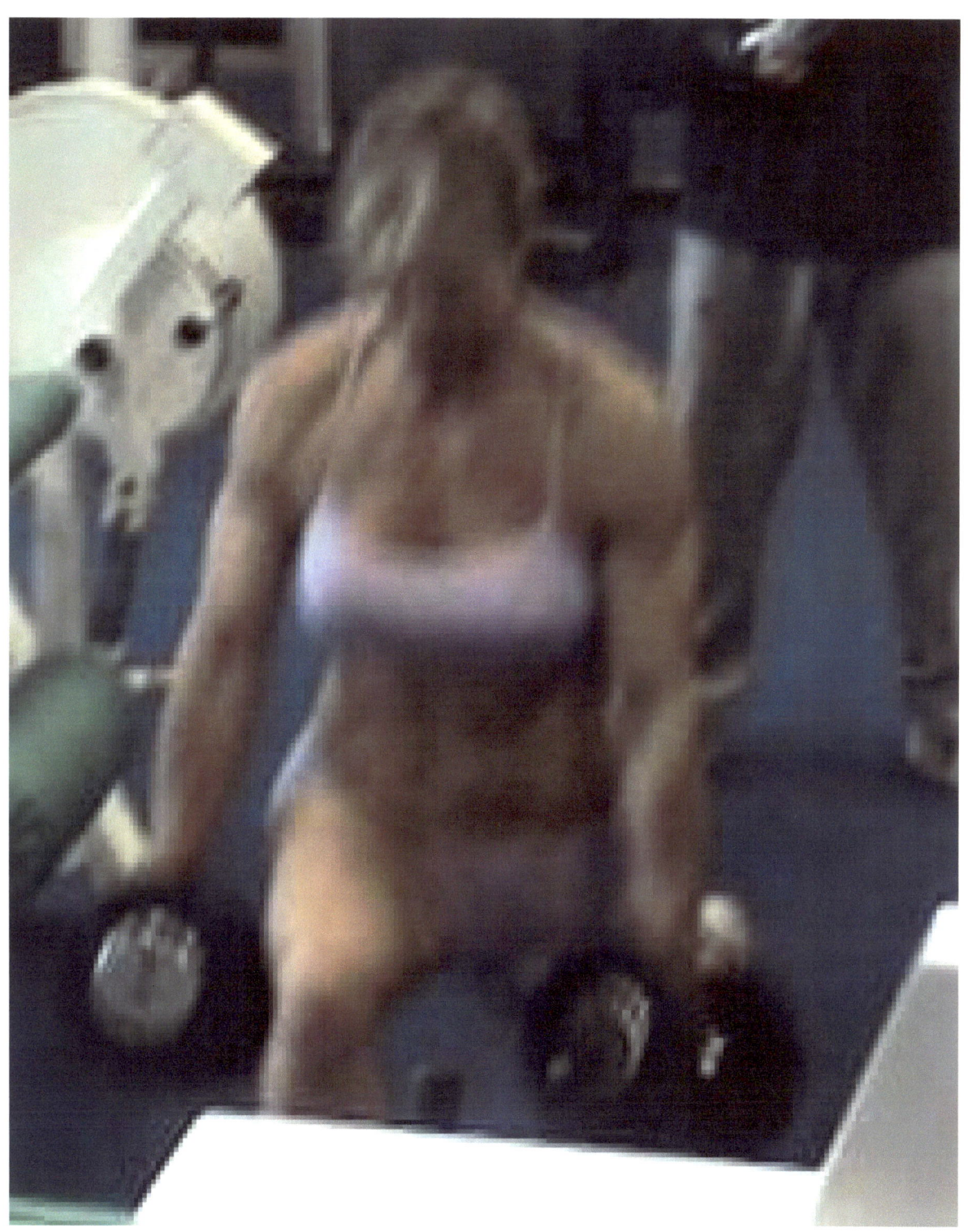

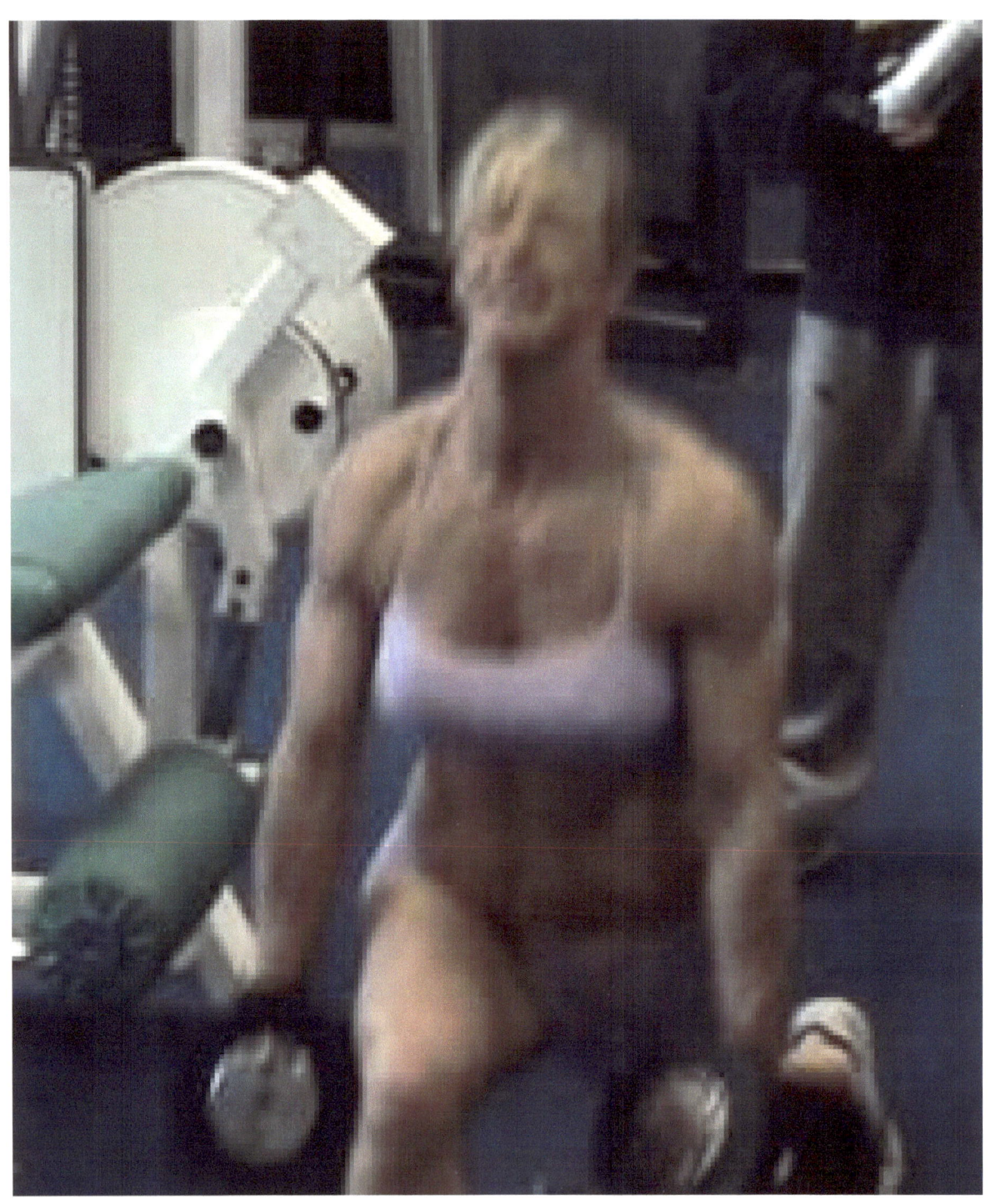

5. Seated Leg Curls & Dumb-bell Straddle squats.

This again pre-exhausts the hamstrings but works the entire glute and thigh area with the straddles squats. This workout really does have to be experienced for its ability to hit the muscle groups in a very unique and unusual way. Three superset straight off. The straddles are worked to failure and are kept under continuous tension. This is a real butt and thigh blasting combination to finish this session with. You will love the results.

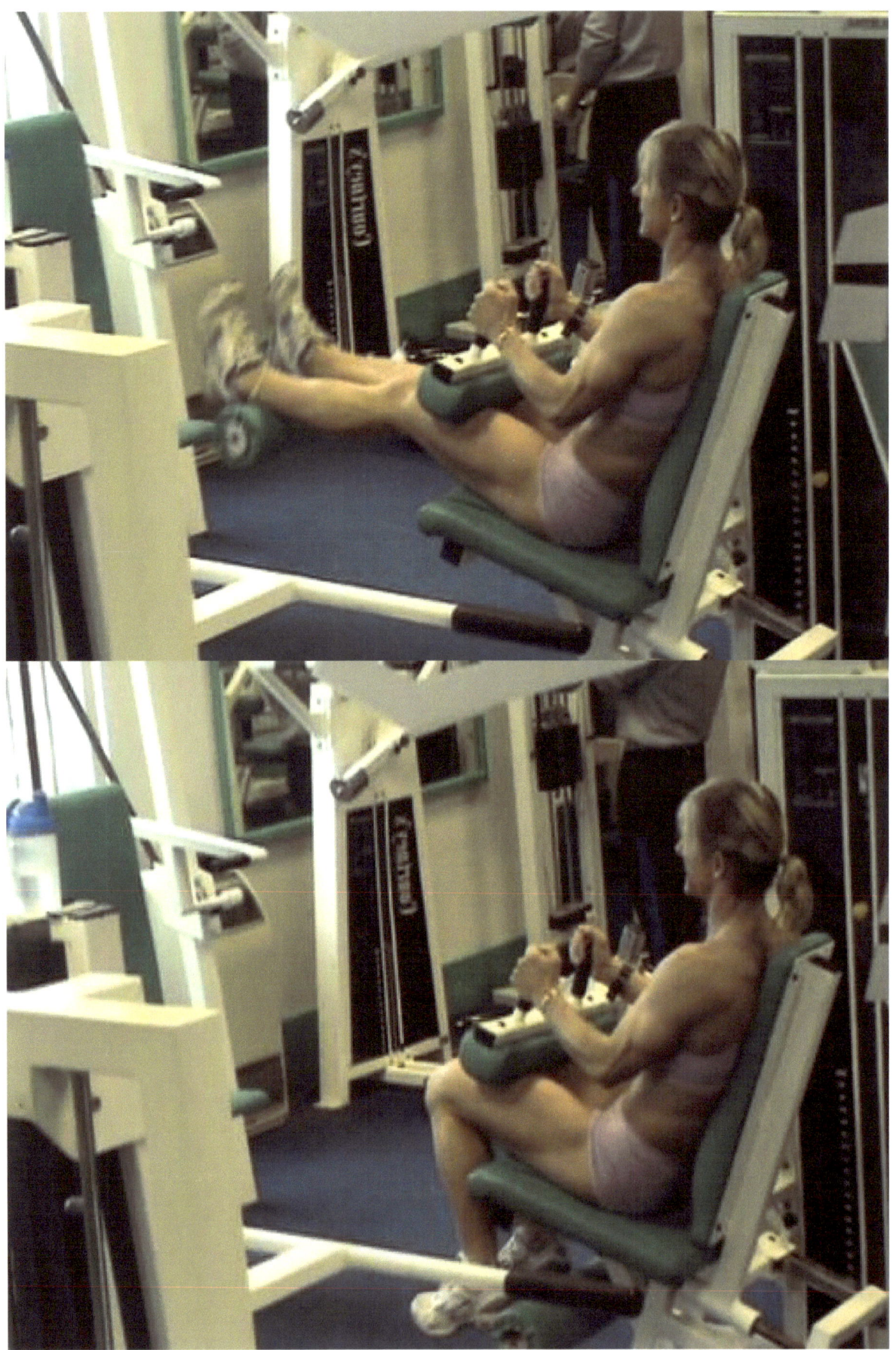

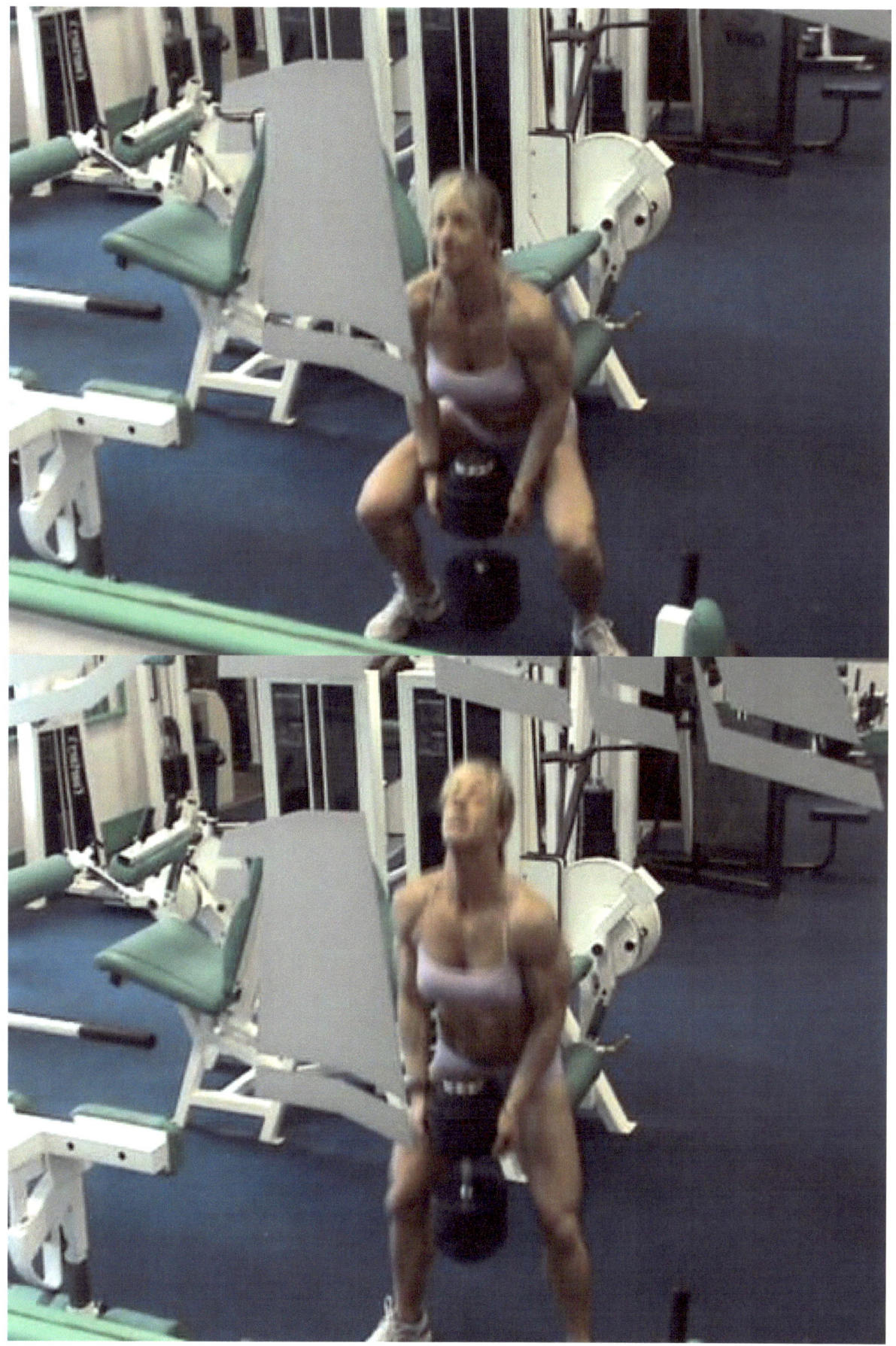

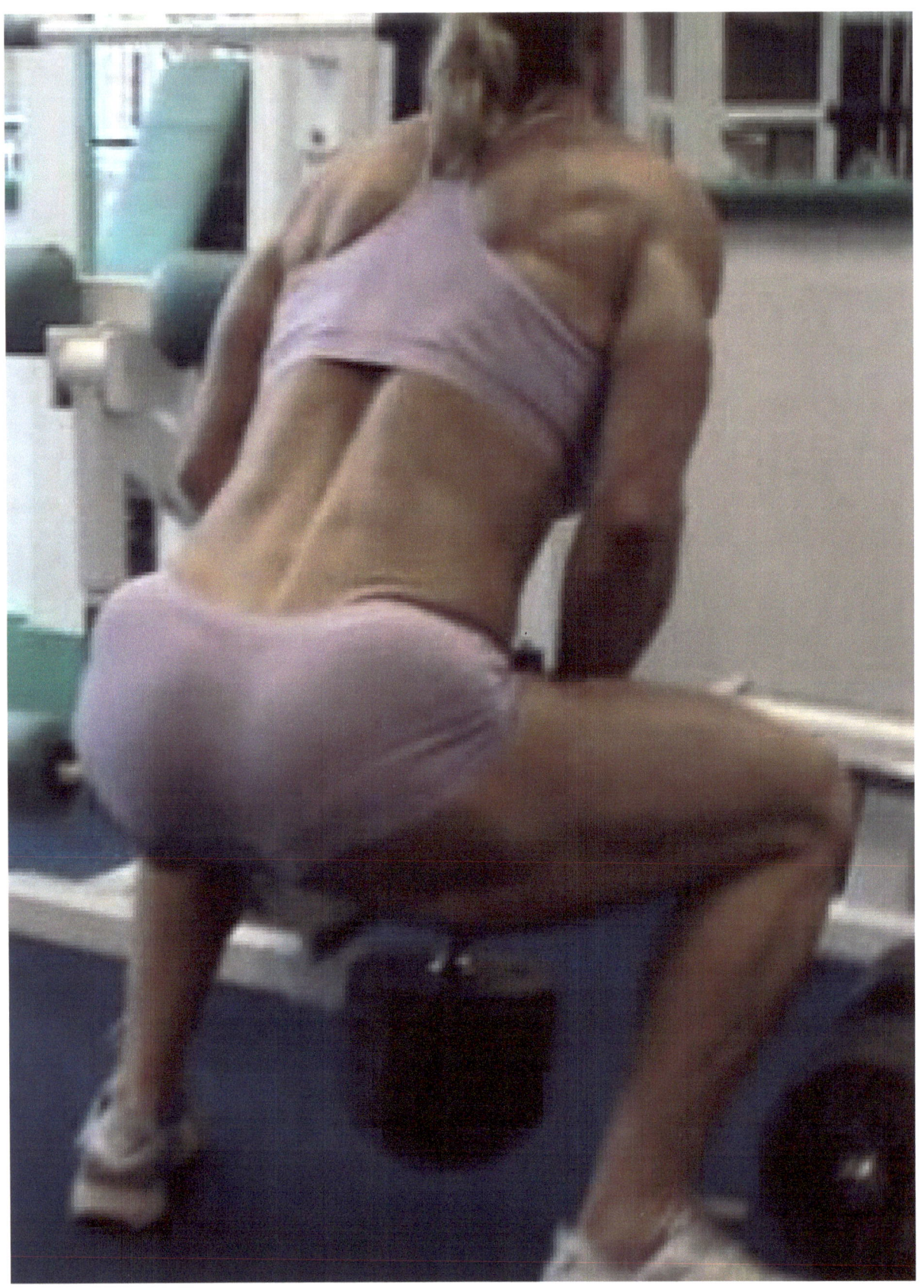

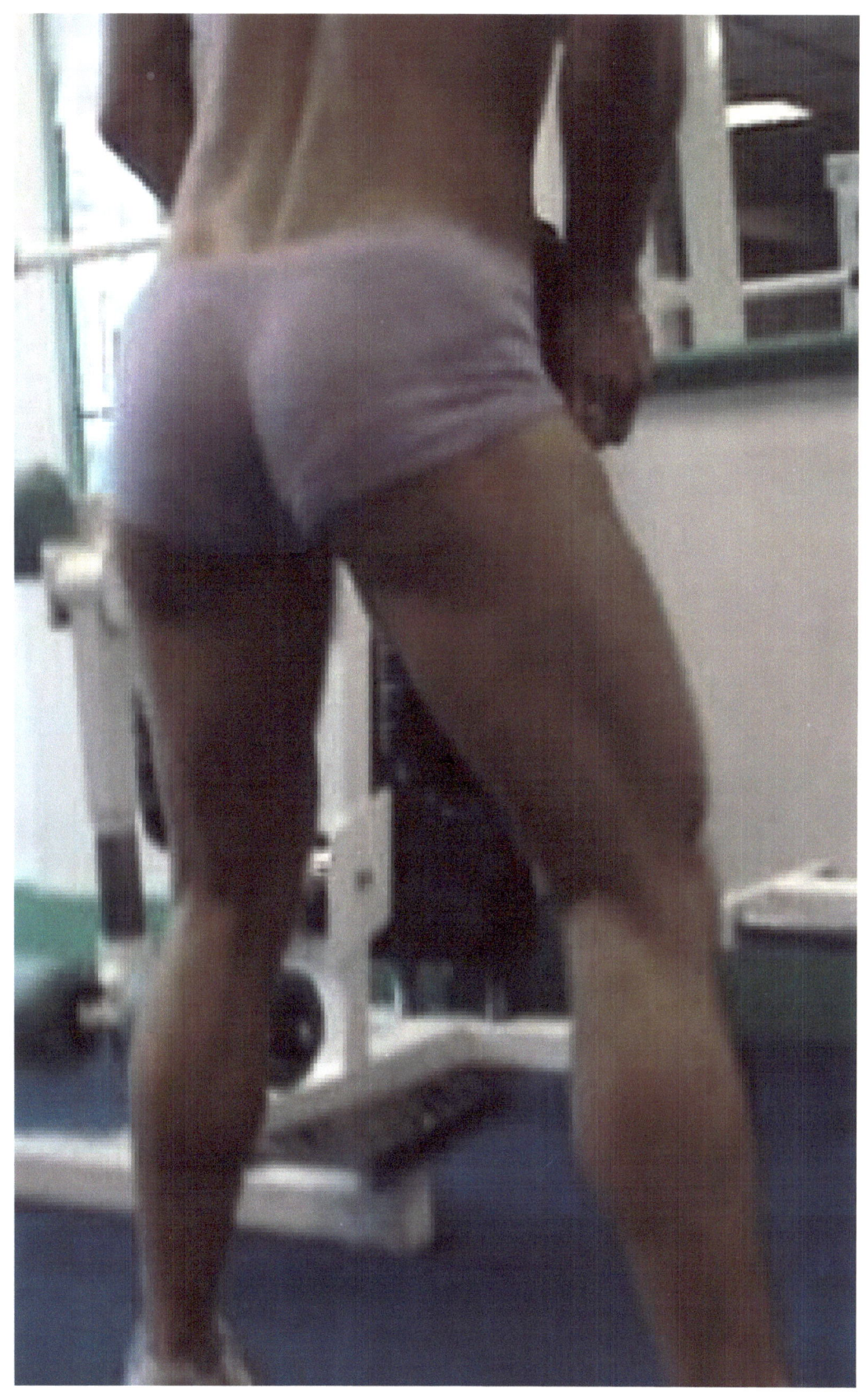

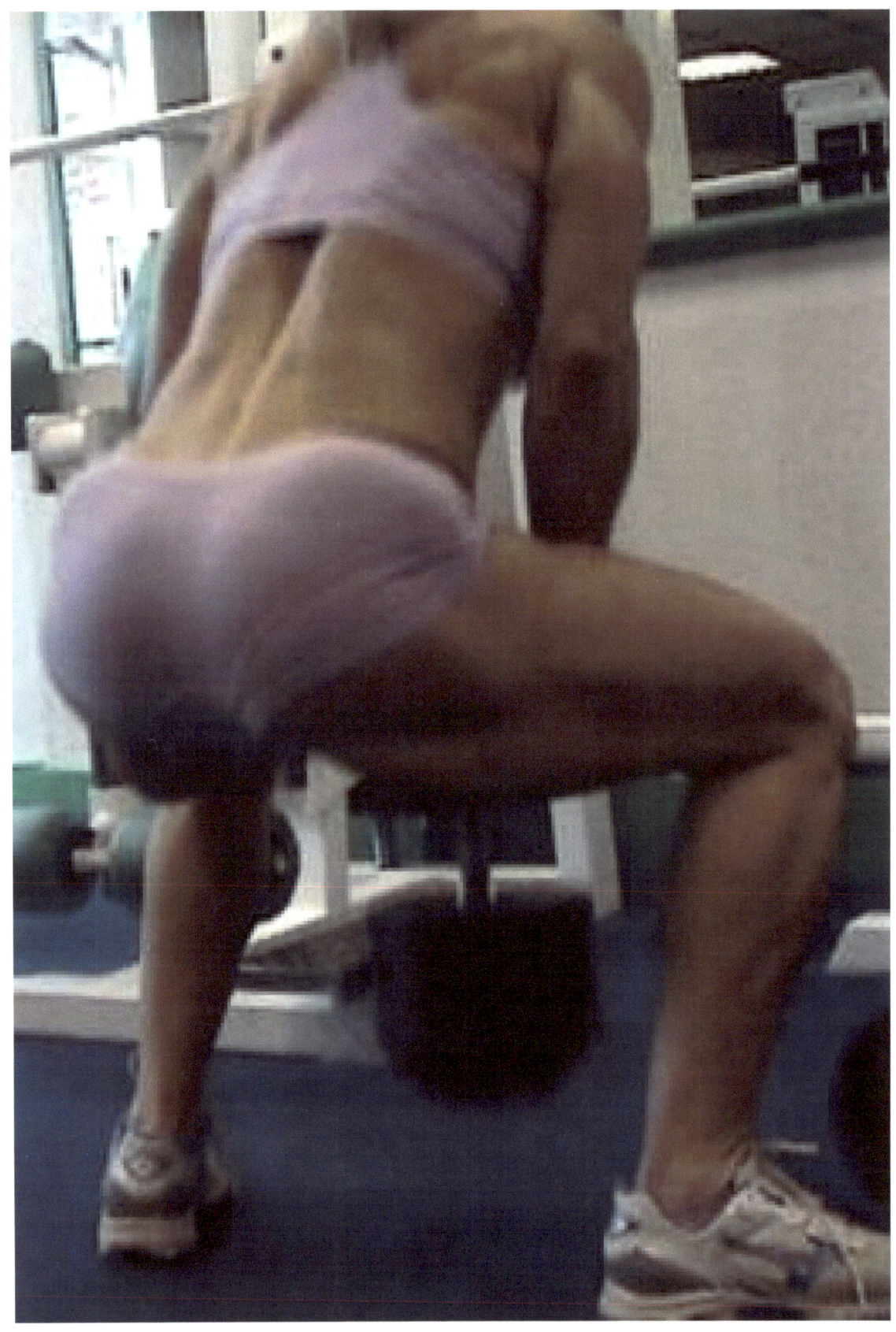

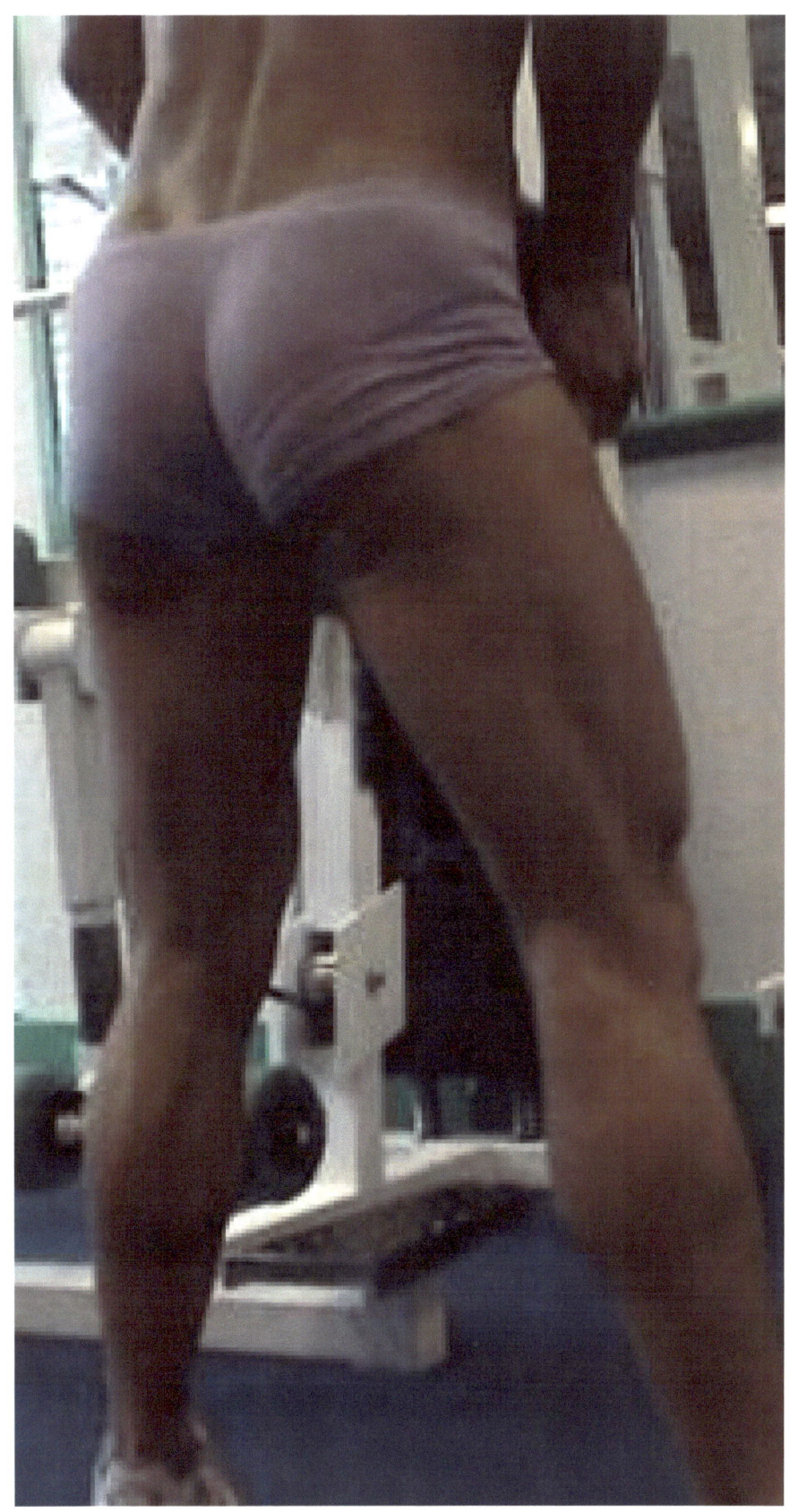

The End

Many thanks

Get In - Work Hard - Get Out

www.ingramcontent.com/pod-product-compliance
Lightning Source LLC
Chambersburg PA
CBHW041533280526
45792CB00004B/1493